ESSENTIAL GUIDE TO IMPETIGO

Everything You Need to Know About Impetigo: Diagnosis, Treatment, and Prevention

DR. CASEY LOREN

DISCLAIMER

This book's content is only meant to be used for general informative purposes. Although the author has taken great care to ensure the content is accurate and thorough, no warranties or assurances on the information's accuracy, correctness, or reliability are provided. It is recommended that readers employ their own judgment and discretion when applying any material found in this book to their particular situation.

The information in this book is not intended to replace professional advice, nor is the author an expert in any of the subjects covered. It is recommended that readers consult with experienced professionals regarding any particular issues or concerns.

Any name that may be mentioned or referred in this book does not imply endorsement, recommendation, or relationship on the part of the author with any person, entity, good, website, or association. These references are made only for informational purposes and are not meant to be taken as recommendations or endorsements.

The information contained in this book may cause readers to suffer loss or damage, for which the author disclaims all obligation and accountability. The only people accountable for the decisions and actions taken by readers using the information presented are themselves.

Any names, characters, companies, locations, activities, occasions, and incidents referenced in this book are either made up or the result of the author's imagination. Any likeness to real people, living or dead, or to real things is entirely coincidental.

This book's content may change at any time, without prior notice, according to the author.

The onus is on the reader to verify whether there have been any updates or revisions.

The reader accepts the conditions of this disclaimer by reading this book. Please do not read this book or use its contents if you do not agree to these terms.

9

CHAPTER 1

OVERVIEW OF IMPETIGO

Red sores or blisters that grow on the hands, face, and other parts of the body are indicative of impetigo, a common bacterial skin illness. It is extremely contagious and typically affects youngsters, however it can also strike adults. Effective management and prevention of impetigo depend on having a thorough understanding of its many facets, including its types, causes, symptoms, diagnosis, risk factors, complications, early detection, treatment choices, and preventive measures.

Impetigo Types

Impetigo comes in two primary varieties: nonbullous and bullous. The most prevalent impetigo is nonbullous, characterized by tiny blisters that rupture and leave a crust with a honey hue. Contrarily, blisters packed with fluid in bullous impetigo are larger and may not rupture as quickly as blisters in nonbullous impetigo.

Impetigo Causes

Bacteria, most frequently Staphylococcus aureus and Streptococcus pyogenes, are the main cause of impetigo. Cuts, bug bites, and other breaches in the skin's protective layer can allow these germs to penetrate the epidermis and cause infection.

Impetigo symptoms

Impetigo is characterized by red, often itchy sores or blisters, enlarged lymph nodes around the affected area, and a distinctive crust that turns honey-colored as the blisters rupture. The blisters in bullous impetigo are bigger and might not rupture as quickly.

Identification of Impetigo

To pinpoint the precise bacteria causing the infection, doctors may also conduct a bacterial culture in addition to diagnosing impetigo based on the look of the skin sores.

Who's in Danger?

Kids are more likely to get impetigo if they are around other people a lot, such as in childcare facilities. Additionally more vulnerable are those with compromised immune systems, skin disorders, or injuries that damage the skin barrier.

Impetigo's Complications

Although impetigo is often a mild and self-limiting illness, if treatment is not received, consequences may include cellulitis, a deeper skin infection, post-streptococcal glomerulonephritis, a kidney ailment, and the infection spreading to other regions of the body.

The Value of Early Identification

To stop the infection from spreading to others and lower the chance of consequences, impetigo must be detected as soon as possible. Early diagnosis and intervention can also reduce symptoms and expedite the healing process.

An Overview of Available Therapies

Topical antibiotics, including mupirocin, are commonly used to treat impetigo by applying them directly to the afflicted skin. Oral antibiotics may be recommended in cases of greater severity or where the infection has spread. It's critical to finish the entire antibiotic course as prescribed by a medical expert.

Preventive Actions

Good hygiene practices, such as routine hand washing, covering cuts and scrapes, avoiding direct contact with infected people, and quickly seeking medical assistance for any signs of infection, are preventive measures against impetigo.

By being aware of these important features of impetigo, people can take preventative measures against infection, identify symptoms early, and seek the right medical attention for efficient treatment.

CHAPTER 2

RECOGNIZING THE BACTERIAL OFFENDERS

Staphylococcus aureus:

This bacterium is frequently found in human nasal passages and on skin. Even though it is usually safe, when it gets into the body through cuts, wounds, or mucous membranes, it can lead to infections. These infections can be anything from simple skin infections like impetigo to more serious illnesses like cellulitis or even infections of the bloodstream. Antibiotic resistance in Staphylococcus aureus is well-known, which might make treatment difficult in some situations.

2. Another bacterium that can cause impetigo is Streptococcus pyogenes, usually referred to as Group A Streptococcus. Numerous illnesses, such as strep throat, scarlet fever, and skin infections like impetigo, are caused by it. Both

respiratory droplets and direct contact with an infected individual can transmit Streptococcus pyogenes. Antibiotic treatment must begin as soon as possible to avoid problems like cellulitis or post-streptococcal glomerulonephritis.

Other Bacterial Infections:

Impetigo can also be caused by germs other than Staphylococcus aureus and Streptococcus pyogenes. These could include Methicillin-resistant Staphylococcus aureus (MRSA), Haemophilus influenzae, and Streptococcus pneumoniae strains. Effective treatment depends on identifying the particular bacteria causing the infection.

Transmission of Bacteria:

Respiratory droplets, contaminated objects or surfaces, or direct touch with an infected person can all spread impetigo-causing bacteria. Hand washing regularly is one example of good hygiene practices that can help stop the spread of bacteria.

5. Several factors, such as temperature, humidity, pH levels, the availability of nutrients, and the presence of competing microorganisms, can influence the growth of bacteria. It's critical to comprehend these elements to stop bacterial infections and stop their spread.

Antibiotic Resistance:

Bacteria can become resistant to antibiotics by developing defense mechanisms, which makes treating infections more challenging. The emergence of resistant bacteria can be attributed to the overuse or misuse of antibiotics. Fighting antibiotic resistance requires proper antibiotic stewardship.

The importance of cleanliness:

Preventing bacterial illnesses like impetigo can be achieved by adhering to basic hygiene habits, which include frequent hand washing with soap and water, covering and cleaning wounds, and not sharing personal objects. Reducing the prevalence of bacterial infections requires educating people about good hygiene habits.

Common Myths:

There are several common misconceptions regarding bacterial infections. These include the notions that all bacteria are dangerous (many bacteria are useful or innocuous) and that antibiotics are always required for treating infections (they are ineffective against viral infections). Promoting acceptable healthcare practices requires educating people to dispel these myths.

Influence of Climate on Bacterial Infections:

The incidence and dissemination of bacterial infections are subject to the influence of climate. Bacteria can survive and spread in response to a variety of environmental factors, including temperature, humidity, and seasonal fluctuations. Comprehending these climate-related variables can facilitate the execution of focused preventive and mitigation strategies.

Recognizing Resistant Strains:

Recognizing resistant bacterial strains, like MRSA, is essential for directing the right antibiotic treatment. To ascertain whether bacteria are susceptible to different antibiotics, laboratory testing is frequently necessary for this. Healthcare professionals need to be on the lookout for new resistant strains and modify treatment plans accordingly.

Healthcare providers and patients alike can have a better understanding of and ability to treat bacterial illnesses such as impetigo by thoroughly addressing these factors.

CHAPTER 3

IMPETIGO'S CLINICAL PRESENTATION

Common Skin Illnesses:

Impetigo typically manifests as tiny, red sores that burst and form crusts the color of honey. Although they can occur anywhere on the body, these lesions are frequently found around the mouth and nose. They are usually not painful, though they could be itchy. Impetigo is distinguished by the distinctive look of the crusts, which also helps with diagnosis.

Unusual Demonstrations:

Impetigo can exhibit itself in unusual ways, while the classic form is honey-colored crusts. These can include eczematous impetigo, which is a more widespread rash mimicking eczema, or enormous bullae filled with clear fluid, known as bullous impetigo. These differences may make diagnosis more difficult and call for a thorough examination.

The distinctions between impetigo that is bullous and non-bullous:

Larger, fluid-filled blisters are more common in bullous impetigo than the smaller, crusted lesions that are seen in non-bullous impetigo. Although the causing bacteria (Streptococcus pyogenes or Staphylococcus aureus) are typically the same, the clinical presentation differs, with bullous impetigo more commonly afflicting newborns and young children.

Impetigo Among Various Age Groups:

While impetigo can afflict people of any age, children—especially those under the age of five—are more likely to contract it. It is frequently linked to other skin disorders or weakened immune systems in adults.

Comprehending age-related trends aids in developing suitable treatment strategies and foreseeing any issues.

How to Identify Secondary Infections

Impetigo that is not well controlled or is left untreated can lead to complications including cellulitis or the development of abscesses. To identify secondary infections early and take appropriate action, it is imperative to keep an eye out for any signs of spreading redness, warmth, discomfort, or systemic symptoms like fever.

Differential diagnosis's importance

For treatment to be effective, impetigo must be distinguished from other skin illnesses such as eczema, herpes simplex virus infections, or fungal infections. For a precise diagnosis and focused treatment, a clinical examination, microbiological testing, and occasionally a histological study may be required.

Evaluating Intensity:

Determining the optimal treatment option for impetigo involves evaluating its severity and extent. Topical antibiotics may be effective in treating mild cases, but oral antibiotics or, in rare situations, hospitalization may be necessary for severe or widespread infections.

Problems to Be Aware of:

Impetigo can lead to complications such as lymphangitis, cellulitis, and post-streptococcal sequelae such as rheumatic fever or acute glomerulonephritis. To avoid these issues and guarantee the best possible results, it is essential to keep an eye out for any indications of systemic involvement or escalating skin problems.

Effects on Patients' Minds:

Impetigo is one example of a skin ailment that can have a serious psychological effect, particularly in young people. Severe lesions, social stigma, and worries about infection might cause shame, anxiety, or low self-esteem. Holistic patient treatment must address these psychosocial factors.

Taking Pictures to Document Progress:

Taking pictures to record the development of impetigo is beneficial for several reasons. It facilitates instructive conversations with patients and caregivers, offers a visual record for tracking response to therapy, and can be used as a resource for upcoming evaluations or consultations.

Healthcare professionals may guarantee comprehensive assessment, precise diagnosis, and efficient therapy of impetigo while taking patients' overall needs into account by addressing these factors in full.

CHAPTER 4

METHODS OF DIAGNOSIS

Visual Inspection

Impetigo is mostly diagnosed by visual examination. Examining the afflicted areas, which are typically the skin, is necessary to look for telltale symptoms like tiny, red, itchy bumps that develop into blisters and eventually turn into a yellow crust.

Swab Encounters

Swab cultures are frequently performed to identify the impetigo-causing bacteria, which are either Streptococcus pyogenes or Staphylococcus aureus. The afflicted area is cleaned with a sterile swab, and the sample is subsequently grown in a lab to determine the precise bacteria.

PCR Examination

Testing with PCR (Polymerase Chain Reaction) is a molecular method for finding bacterial DNA. In cases of impetigo, it can assist confirm the presence of Staphylococcus aureus or Streptococcus pyogenes by providing quick and precise results.

Procedures for Biopsies

A biopsy might be carried out in specific situations where the diagnosis is not apparent or if there are complications. A microscopic examination of a small sample of skin tissue is performed to determine the degree of infection or to rule out other skin disorders.

Standards for Differential Diagnosis

Differential diagnosis is the process of separating impetigo from other skin diseases such as ringworm, herpes simplex virus, and eczema. An accurate diagnosis is made by taking into account factors like the appearance of lesions, the patient's medical history, and the outcomes of laboratory tests.

The Value of a Correct Diagnosis

To start the right therapy for impetigo as soon as possible, an accurate diagnosis is essential. A misdiagnosis may result in inadequate therapy and unfavorable outcomes including infection transmission or resistance to antibiotics.

It is advisable to visit a dermatologist or infectious disease specialist in difficult instances or when routine therapies are not working. Experts can provide cutting-edge methods of diagnosis, customized treatment plans, and patient care strategies.

Diagnostic Test Restrictions

It's critical to remember that no diagnostic procedure is flawless. Even though they are useful, PCR testing and swab cultures can occasionally produce false-positive or false-negative results. When interpreting test results, clinical judgment and linkage with patient symptoms are crucial.

Interpreting the Outcomes

Clinical knowledge is necessary to interpret the outcomes of diagnostic tests. Swab culture or PCR test findings that are positive confirm the impetigo diagnosis; nevertheless, negative results do not completely rule it out. Interpreting the results requires taking into account the patient's history, physical examination findings, and therapy response.

Additional Testing

To evaluate the effectiveness of the treatment and make sure the impetigo completely resolves, follow-up testing could be required. Recurrence or problems can be avoided by doing PCR testing or repeat swab cultures to verify bacterial eradication.

Healthcare practitioners can effectively identify and treat impetigo by incorporating certain diagnostic approaches and factors, which will enhance patient outcomes.

CHAPTER 5
METHODS OF TREATMENT

Topical Antibiotics:

The first line of treatment for impetigo is frequently topical antibiotics. They are applied directly to the skin's afflicted areas and come in ointment or cream form. Topical antibiotics like retapamulin and mupirocin are frequently used to treat impetigo. These drugs function by eradicating the infection-causing microorganisms. It's critical to adhere to your doctor's recommendations about the frequency and duration of antibiotic application.

Oral Antibiotics:

Oral antibiotics may be recommended in more severe instances or when impetigo has spread widely. These antibiotics, which include dicloxacillin and cephalexin, combat the infection from within the body by acting systemically. When topical therapies alone are insufficient or when there is a risk of complications like cellulitis, oral antibiotics are often saved for certain situations.

Combination Therapies:

For a more intensive course of treatment, topical and oral antibiotics may occasionally be used in combination. This method is frequently used when the infection is pervasive, recurring, or unresponsive to previous therapies. Combining various medicines can improve the way they target the bacteria and lower the chance that they will become resistant to them.

Wound Care Procedures:

Managing impetigo requires proper wound care. This entails keeping the afflicted regions dry and clean, refraining from picking or scratching the lesions, and, if required, covering them with sterile bandages. To promote speedier healing, gently wash the area with soap and water to help remove any crusts or debris.

Importance of Compliance:

Adherence to prescribed regimens is essential for the effective therapy of impetigo. This entails doing as directed by your healthcare professional about the use of medications, the length of treatment, and any extra wound care procedures. Medication omissions or early treatment discontinuation can result in insufficient healing and possible infection recurrence.

Handling Allergic responses:

Although they are rare, allergic responses to topical medicines or antibiotics might happen. It's critical to recognize any symptoms of an allergic reaction, like rash, itching, swelling, or trouble breathing, and to get medical assistance as soon as possible if they do. If an allergic reaction is suspected, your healthcare professional can modify your treatment plan.

Alternative Medical Treatments:

For impetigo, some people may investigate complementary and alternative medical treatments including essential oils or herbal medicines. These methods may be supported by anecdotal evidence, but there hasn't been much research done on their efficacy or safety while treating impetigo. Before utilizing alternative therapies, it is imperative to speak with a healthcare provider to be sure they are safe and work well with traditional treatments.

Effectiveness of Home Remedies:

While some home treatments, such as warm compresses or diluted vinegar soaks, may relieve impetigo symptoms, they shouldn't be used in place of medical care. They can support conventional treatments, but they shouldn't take the place of prescription drugs or wound care procedures.

Importance of Prompt Treatment:

To avoid consequences and minimize the infection's spread to others, impetigo must be treated promptly. The likelihood of repeated episodes can be reduced and symptoms can be resolved more quickly with the prompt use of antibiotics and strict adherence to treatment regimens.

Handling Repeated Cases:

To determine the underlying causes of recurrent impetigo episodes, a more comprehensive assessment may be necessary. This could involve looking for skin diseases like dermatitis or eczema that predispose people to the infection or analyzing environmental factors that might be promoting bacterial colonization. To stop recurrences, maintenance therapy or long-term preventive measures may be advised in some situations.

CHAPTER 6

PREVENTIVE TECHNIQUES

Personal Cleaning Routines:

• Promote frequent hand washing with soap and water, particularly after handling contaminated objects or spaces.

• Towels, razors, and clothing are examples of personal goods that should not be shared as they can spread the virus.

• Instruct patients on adequate wound care to stop wounds and scratches from spreading impetigo.

Environmental Sanitation:

• Maintain sanitized and clean common areas, including doorknobs and countertops that are often touched.

• Regularly wash towels, bedding, and clothes in hot water with detergent.

• Immediately wash and sanitize toys, particularly in environments used for child care.

Precautions for Isolation:

• Suggest that people suffering from impetigo stay away from close contact with others until the infection has healed or has been cleared by a medical professional.

• To stop the germs from spreading, give sick people different towels and sheets.

Antimicrobial Goods:

• If prescribed by a medical practitioner, take into consideration applying topical antibiotic creams or ointments to cure impetigo.

• Although simple soap and water work well most of the time, use antibacterial soaps when washing your hands.

Vaccination-Related Considerations:

• Although there isn't a specific vaccination for impetigo at this time, following national vaccination guidelines and staying up to date on immunizations might help people avoid other infections that could put them at risk for impetigo.

Initiatives for Community Education:

• Provide instructional resources for community settings that address impetigo transmission, prevention, and treatment.

• Hold lectures or workshops to spread knowledge and encourage good hygiene habits.

Early Intervention Programs:

• Urge anyone who observes signs of impetigo, such as blisters that ooze and crust or red sores, to get medical help right once.

- Educate medical professionals on how to appropriately identify and diagnose impetigo.

Schools' and daycares' roles:

• Put in place procedures that require afflicted kids to stay home from daycare or school until they are cleared by a medical professional or until they are no longer contagious.

• Inform parents and employees about techniques for preventing impetigo.

Consciousness in Medical Environments:

• Verify that infection control procedures are followed by healthcare facilities to stop the spread of impetigo among personnel and patients.

• Teach medical personnel how to properly diagnose and treat impetigo.

Including Prevention in Everyday Activities:

• Motivate people and families to incorporate good hygiene habits into their everyday lives, such as frequent hand washing and dressing and cleaning of wounds.

• Offer incentives and reminders to ensure regular adherence to preventative measures.

Effective impetigo prevention can be achieved by addressing each of these preventive techniques in-depth and implementing them into everyday activities and community initiatives.

CHAPTER 7

EFFECTS ON PARTICULAR POPULATIONS

Children's Impetigo

Children are more likely to get impetigo when they are between the ages of two and five. Usually, it starts as red sores around the mouth and nose that soon develop into blisters before crusting over. Due to close contact, children in childcare or school environments are particularly vulnerable.

Topical antibiotics are usually used as a form of treatment, though in more serious cases, oral antibiotics can be required. Crucial preventive actions include maintaining clean, hygienic conditions, refraining from itching and practicing proper hygiene.

Adult Impetigo

Although impetigo is more frequent in children, it can also strike adults, particularly in those with immune-suppressive disorders or those who have close contact with infected people. Red lesions that develop into blisters and crust over resemble those seen in youngsters.

Adult patients with impetigo might need to take stronger antibiotics or finish their treatment more slowly. It takes good hygiene habits, including frequent hand washing, to stop the infection from spreading.

Impetigo in Senior Individuals

Impetigo can occur in elderly individuals because of compromised immune systems, brittle skin, and close quarters, especially in long-term care facilities. While the illness may present similarly to those in other age groups, underlying medical issues may make it more difficult to treat.

For older individuals, careful management is essential to preventing complications like cellulitis or systemic infection. This includes adequate antibiotic therapy and gentle cleansing of afflicted regions.

Impetigo in People with Reduced Immune Systems

Severe impetigo and associated sequelae are more common in people with weakened immune systems, such as those with HIV/AIDS, cancer patients, and those on immunosuppressive medicines. The illness could spread quickly and need intensive care. When treating impetigo in immunocompromised patients, timely introduction of appropriate antibiotics and close supervision by medical personnel are crucial to preventing future problems.

Pregnancy-Related Issues

When impetigo develops during pregnancy, especially around the time of delivery, it might be worrisome. There may be worries regarding infection transfer during labor even though the infection itself is typically not dangerous to the fetus.

Those who have impetigo during pregnancy should consult a doctor right away to get the right care and avoid any difficulties for both the mother and the unborn child.

Effects on Emotional Well-Being

The psychological effects of having impetigo can be profound, particularly for those who suffer from severe or recurrent episodes. A visible infection might cause feelings of humiliation, worry, or despair in addition to possible social stigma.

People with impetigo can manage the emotional components of the condition with the assistance of healthcare experts, education about the condition, and access to mental health resources.

Misconceptions and Social Stigma

Sometimes people misinterpret impetigo, which results in misconceptions and social stigma. Individuals could mistakenly think it's the outcome of bad hygiene or connect it to other unfavorable associations.

Public awareness campaigns and education initiatives can help debunk misconceptions about impetigo, lessen stigma, and advance knowledge of the infection's causes and remedies.

Assistance for Nurses

Effective management of impetigo infection may necessitate support and direction for caregivers, particularly in vulnerable groups such as children or the elderly. This covers using appropriate hygiene procedures, giving prescriptions, and spotting warning indications of problems.

To guarantee the best possible care and stop the spread of impetigo in contexts where caregivers are present, healthcare providers can provide information and tools to caregivers.

Resolving Vulnerable Groups' Concerns

Impetigo treatment may be more difficult for vulnerable populations, such as those who live in cramped housing or have limited access to healthcare. A multimodal strategy including community organizations, public health campaigns, and healthcare practitioners is needed to address these issues.

The effects of impetigo can be lessened by initiatives to increase access to healthcare, encourage good hygiene, and offer specialized assistance to communities that are particularly at risk.

Promoting Access to Fair Healthcare

Promoting fair access to healthcare services for impetigo sufferers is essential, particularly for those living in underprivileged areas. This entails promoting outreach initiatives, culturally competent treatment, and reasonably priced pharmaceuticals.

Working together, advocacy organizations, legislators, and healthcare professionals may advance laws and programs that guarantee everyone, regardless of background or situation, equitable access to healthcare.

CHAPTER 8
INVESTIGATION AND ORIGINALITY

contemporary Research Trends:

Understanding the epidemiology, risk factors, etiology, and treatment effects of impetigo is a major focus of contemporary research. Numerous bacteria, such as Streptococcus pyogenes and Staphylococcus aureus, are being studied for their potential roles in the development of impetigo. Researchers are also looking into how antibiotic use, hygiene habits, and socioeconomic factors affect the prevalence and recurrence rates of impetigo.

Vaccine Development:

Research is currently being done to produce a vaccine to prevent impetigo. Researchers are looking into antigen targets that can trigger immune responses that defend against the impetigo-causing bacteria. Preclinical and clinical trials are being conducted on vaccine candidates to evaluate their safety, effectiveness, and potential for broad use in populations at risk.

Novel Techniques for Treatment:

To tackle issues like antibiotic resistance and treatment failure, novel techniques for treating impetigo are being investigated. These methods include systemic treatments like oral antibiotics and immunomodulators, as well as topical ones like new antibacterial medicines and immune-modulating substances. Interventions using complementary and alternative medicine are also being studied.

Studies on antibiotic Resistance:

One major worry is the increase in antibiotic resistance in bacteria that cause impetigo. The main goals of research are to find novel drug targets, comprehend the mechanisms underlying resistance, and create countermeasures. This involves surveillance initiatives to track trends in resistance and encourage the prudent use of antibiotics.

Public health initiatives:

Through immunization campaigns, hygiene promotion, and education, public health initiatives seek to prevent and control impetigo. Enhancing access to healthcare services is another goal of these programs, particularly in impoverished areas where impetigo prevalence may be higher. Effective public health measures require cooperation between community organizations, legislators, and healthcare professionals.

Global Impetigo Burden:

The prevalence of impetigo varies greatly among people and geographical areas, with lower- and middle-income nations showing the highest rates. Epidemiological studies, burden-of-disease assessments, and economic evaluations are among the research methods used to measure the global impetigo burden to determine the impact on society and healthcare systems.

The use of telemedicine for remote consultations, electronic health records for patient management, and diagnostic instruments for quick and precise identification of impetigo infections are just a few examples of how technology is vital to the management of impetigo. Digital platforms and mobile health apps also help with patient education and treatment regimen adherence.

Patient-centered Research:

To better understand patients' experiences, preferences, and priorities about diagnosis, treatment, and outcomes, patient-centered research on impetigo is conducted. The creation of collaborative decision-making techniques, individualized care plans, and support services to enhance patient happiness and treatment compliance are all influenced by the findings of this research.

Future Expectations:

Novel medicines that target particular pathogenic processes, vaccine development advancements, and precision medicine strategies based on individual risk profiles are all anticipated developments in impetigo research. It is anticipated that advancements in the knowledge and treatment of impetigo will come from interdisciplinary partnerships, collaborative research networks, and data-sharing programs.

Advocacy for Funding and Support:

To ensure that impetigo research, education, and healthcare services receive the funding and support they need, advocacy is essential. In addition to advocating for laws that support infection prevention and antibiotic stewardship, advocates also try to increase public awareness of the effects of impetigo and mobilize resources to address unmet needs in impetigo management. Encouraging organizations, researchers, legislators, and industry stakeholders must work together to keep impetigo research and innovation moving forward.

CHAPTER 9

RESOURCES AND PATIENT EDUCATION

Making Materials for Patient Information

The fundamentals of impetigo, including its causes, symptoms, risk factors, diagnosis, available treatments, and preventative measures, should be covered in patient education materials. Diagrams and other visual aids can be useful in helping to clarify concepts. A friendly tone, understandable explanations, and clear language can improve readability and engagement.

Online Communities and Support Groups

By putting patients and caregivers in touch with online forums and support groups, impetigo management strategies, shared experiences, and important emotional support can be obtained. These platforms can also serve as resources for newly available treatments, updated information, and coping mechanisms for condition-related difficulties.

dependable internet sources

A list of trustworthy websites, including government health portals, respectable medical websites, and the websites of professional associations, should be curated to guarantee that patients and caregivers have access to current and accurate information regarding impetigo. The significance of confirming information from reliable sources must be emphasized to prevent disinformation.

Teaching Caretakers

Teaching caregivers about impetigo entails educating them on the illness's causes, symptoms, available treatments, and preventative measures. Through this instruction, caregivers will be more equipped to identify the early indicators of impetigo, seek the necessary medical attention, and administer care at home. It's critical to address any worries or inquiries caregivers might have and give them access to resources for more help.

Workplace and School Guidelines

Creating policies for businesses and educational institutions about impetigo can assist stop the infection's spread and guarantee everyone is in a safe environment. These standards might cover things like best practices for personal hygiene, measures to exclude affected people from social situations, and methods for sanitizing shared areas. Effective implementation and enforcement of these principles necessitate cooperation with employers and school administrations.

Advocacy Organizations

Partnering with advocacy groups that address infectious diseases or skin health issues can help spread the word about impetigo, encourage research projects, and push for better treatment access for those who are afflicted. These groups may also provide community outreach initiatives, educational resources, and support services.

Obtaining Reasonably Priced Care

Encouraging insurance coverage, promoting generic pharmaceuticals, and supporting programs that offer financial assistance to persons with little resources are all necessary to ensure that impetigo patients have access to cheap treatment. Addressing obstacles to treatment access can be facilitated by cooperation with pharmaceutical firms, advocacy organizations, and healthcare providers.

Programs for Financial Assistance

People with impetigo can obtain essential medications and treatments without financial hardship by identifying and supporting financial assistance programs, such as patient assistance programs, pharmaceutical discount programs, and government assistance efforts. Effective condition management can be greatly improved by informing patients and caregivers about these programs and helping them with the application process.

Culturally Sensitive education

When delivering impetigo education, it is important to take into account cultural attitudes, behaviors, and beliefs toward wellness and health. Developing instructional materials, outreach initiatives, and communication tactics that are culturally sensitive can improve comprehension, participation, and treatment and prevention adherence.

Encouraging Patients to Speak Up for Their Rights

Encouraging patients to actively participate in healthcare decisions, teaching them about their rights, and providing them with resources and skills for self-advocacy are all part of empowering patients to speak out for themselves. This includes instructing patients on how to ask questions, get second views, and access support services in addition to communicating with medical professionals. Promoting a team approach to treatment gives patients the ability to actively manage their impetigo and general health.